Trim Your Tummy

A Step-by-Step Manual for Reducing Belly Fat for absolute beginners

Simone Peterson

Chapter One

Trim Your Tummy
What exactly is belly fat?

Visceral fat, also referred to as belly fat, is fat that is stored deep within the abdominal cavity around important-t organs such as the pancreas, liver, and intestines. Visceral fat is more dangerous for your health than subcutaneous fat because it is closer to internal organs than subcutaneous fat is.

To put it briefly, reducing health risks and enhancing general well-being require an awareness of and ability to manage belly fat. Understanding and managing

belly fat is very important for
mitigating health risk and
improving well being

distinguishing Between Visceral and Subcutaneous Fat

Subcutaneous Fat: Beneath the Skin,

• **Location:** Found covering the surface of the body just beneath the skin.

• **Appearance:** Typically jiggly and squishy.

• **Function:** Provides protection and cushioning for underlying tissues and organs, as well as insulation and temperature regulation.

• **Amount:** Although it varies from person to person, subcutaneous fat typically builds up in the abdomen, thighs, hips, and buttocks.

- **Health Implications:** Although it is less strongly associated with metabolic abnormalities than visceral fat, excess subcutaneous fat may nonetheless have a role in obesity-related health disorders.

Visceral Fat: Fat Around Internal Organs

- **Location:** Surrounding internal organs including the liver, pancreas, and intestines, deep within the abdominal cavity.

- **Appearance:** It is internal and not immediately felt; it is not visible from the outside.

- **Function:** Helps produce hormones and regulate metabolism; however, too much visceral fat can interfere with these functions and cause health issues.

- **Amount**: Excess visceral fat is linked to central obesity and can be present in those with a normal BMI as well.

- **Health Implications:** Unlike subcutaneous fat, visceral fat provides greater health risks due to its metabolic activity and proximity to key organs. It is strongly associated to metabolic syndrome, insulin resistance, type 2 diabetes, heart disease, and certain malignancies.

In conclusion, visceral fat is more dangerous for health because it is linked to metabolic problems and a higher risk of chronic diseases, even if subcutaneous fat also plays a role in overall body composition.

significance of Losing Belly Fat for Health and Well-Being

1.Reduce Risk of Chronic Diseases: People who have excess belly fat, especially visceral fat, have a higher chance of developing chronic illnesses like heart disease, type 2 diabetes, and some types of cancer. By losing belly fat, people can lessen their chance of acquiring these dangerous illnesses.

2.Improve Metabolic Health:
Losing belly fat can help people become more insulin sensitive, less inflammatory, and at lower risk of developing metabolic syndrome, which is a collection of disorders that includes elevated blood pressure, high blood sugar, and abnormal cholesterol levels. Belly fat is metabolically active and produces hormones and inflammatory substances that can disrupt metabolic processes.

3. Improved Cardiovascular Health: Reducing belly fat can help improve cardiovascular health by lowering the risk of heart disease and stroke as well

as high blood pressure, elevated
cholesterol, and arterial stiffness,
which are cardiovascular risk
factors.

4. Better Blood Sugar Control:
Reducing belly fat helps people
become more insulin sensitive
and better control their blood
sugar levels, which lower their
risk of type 2 diabetes and its
complications. Insulin resistance
is a condition in which cells
become less responsive to insulin,
resulting in elevated blood sugar
levels.

5. Better Body Composition:
Reducing belly fat and
encouraging muscle growth
through exercise and strength

training can help people achieve a healthier body composition, which is linked to enhanced physical function and general well-being. Excess belly fat can also change body composition by raising the ratio of fat to lean muscle mass.

6. Improved Psychological Well-Being: Having extra abdominal fat can have detrimental psychological impacts, such as low self-worth, problems with body image, and more stress. Reducing belly fat and reaching a healthier weight can boost mental health, self-assurance, and overall quality of life.

Chapter Three

An explanation of the various forms of body fat

1. Subcutaneous fat

• **Location:** Underneath the skin everywhere on the body, but especially in the thighs, hips, buttocks, and abdomen.

• **Appearance:** Visible as pinch able fat, soft and jiggly.

• **Function:** Provides protection and cushioning for underlying tissues and organs, as well as insulation and temperature regulation.

• **Health Implications:**

Although excess subcutaneous fat increases body weight overall, it is generally less metabolically active than visceral fat and has a less correlation with long-term illnesses and metabolic disorders.

2. Visceral fat

• **Location:** Surrounding internal organs including the liver, pancreas, and intestines, deep within the abdominal cavity.

• **Appearance:** It is internal and not immediately felt; it is not visible from the outside.

• **Function:** Helps produce hormones and regulate metabolism; however, too much visceral fat can interfere with these functions and cause health issues.

• **Health Implications:** Because

of its metabolic activity and close proximity to important organs, visceral fat provides significant health risks. It is strongly associated with metabolic syndrome, insulin resistance, type 2 diabetes, heart disease, and certain malignancies.

3. Brown Fat

• **Location:** Small deposits are seen all over the body, particularly in the back, shoulders, and neck.

• **Appearance:** It has a brown tint due to the presence of more iron and mitochondria.

• **Function:** Produces heat by burning calories to keep the body temperature stable, especially when exposed to cold temperatures.

- **Health Implications:** Brown fat activation may help control body weight and may offer treatment benefits for obesity and related disorders. It has been linked to higher energy expenditure and better metabolic health.

4. White Amount of Fat:

- **Location:** Found in visceral and subcutaneous depots as well as other parts of the body.

- **Appearance:** Usually has a whitish or yellowish appearance.

- **Function:** Acts as a store of calories for the body to use when there is an energy shortage by storing energy as triglycerides.

- **Health Implications:** An excess of white fat, especially visceral fat, is linked to insulin resistance, metabolic disorders, and a higher chance of developing chronic illnesses.
It is crucial to comprehend the many forms of body fat, their functions, and the consequences they carry in order to manage weight, promote metabolic health, and lower the risk of diseases linked to obesity.

Factors and Causes of the accumulation of Belly Fat

1. Body type and genetics:

• A person's genetic predisposition can affect where and how fat is deposited in the body, particularly the propensity for fat to build up around the abdomen.

• Compared to people with pear shapes, those with apple shapes typically store more fat around their abdomens.

2. Food Routines:

• Diets high in calories that are high in processed foods, sweets, and bad fats can cause the buildup of belly fat.

• Consuming refined carbohydrates, sugary drinks, and fried foods in excess might encourage weight gain, particularly in the middle.

3. Lack of Physical Exercise:

• A sedentary lifestyle and insufficient exercise on a regular basis can cause an imbalance between calorie intake and expenditure, which can contribute to weight gain and the formation of belly fat.

• Lack of exercise lowers metabolism and muscle mass, which makes weight gain easier, especially around the abdomen.

4. Cortisol and Stress Levels:

• Prolonged stress can raise the stress hormone cortisol production, which encourages fat storage, especially in the abdomen.

• Increased levels of cortisol can increase appetite, which can result in overindulgence and weight gain, with a propensity for the accumulation of fat around the abdomen.

5. Lack of Sleep:

• Hormone balance can be upset by getting too little or poor quality sleep, especially when it comes to hormones that control hunger and metabolism.

• Lack of sleep can cause cravings for high-calorie foods, an increase in appetite, and changes in insulin sensitivity, all of which can contribute to the buildup of belly fat.

6. Alcohol consumption:

• Due to its high calorie content and ability to interfere with metabolism, excessive alcohol use can lead to the buildup of belly fat.

• When alcohol is digested, acetate is produced. The body uses acetate first when producing energy, which causes fat to accumulate, particularly around the abdomen.

7. Hormonal Changes and Aging

• Aging-related hormonal changes, such as decreased testosterone and estrogen levels, might impact metabolism and fat distribution, resulting in a rise in the deposit of fat in the abdomen. Women who are going through menopause frequently see changes in their body composition, with a propensity to accumulate extra fat around their abdomens.

8. Medical Disorders and Drugs:

• Because of hormonal imbalances, a number of medical illnesses, including Cushing's syndrome and polycystic ovarian syndrome (PCOS), can aggravate abdominal obesity.

• As a side effect, some drugs, including corticosteroids and some antidepressants, can also encourage weight gain and the buildup of belly fat.

Chapter Four

Health Dangers of Having Too Much Belly Fat

1. Condition of the Heart:

• There is a clear link between having too much belly fat and a higher risk of cardiovascular conditions like heart disease and stroke.

• Increased levels of cholesterol and triglycerides, arterial stiffness, and inflammation are all associated with belly fat, especially visceral fat, and are risk factors for cardiovascular events.

2. Diabetes type 2:

• Excess belly fat, or abdominal

obesity, is a significant risk factor for type 2 diabetes.

• Hormones and inflammatory chemicals released by visceral fat can hinder the effects of insulin and cause Insulin resistance, which is a prelude to type 2 diabetes.

3. Metabolic Disorder:

• One of the main causes of metabolic syndrome, a collection of illnesses that also includes insulin resistance, high blood pressure, raised blood sugar, and abnormal cholesterol levels, is excess belly fat.

A person with metabolic syndrome has a notably higher risk of heart disease, stroke, and type 2 diabetes.

4. Resistance to Insulin:

• Because visceral fat has an active metabolism, it releases inflammatory chemicals and fatty acids that can disrupt insulin signaling and worsen insulin resistance.

• The body's capacity to control blood sugar levels is hampered by insulin resistance, which raises blood glucose levels and increases the risk of type 2 diabetes.

5. Cancer

• Obesity-related diseases such as colon cancer, breast cancer in women, and prostate cancer in men have been associated with

excess abdominal fat, especially
visceral fat.

• Hormones and growth factors
produced by adipose tissue can
encourage the development and
spread of tumors.

6. Hepatic illness:

• Non-alcoholic fatty liver disease
(NAFLD), a disorder marked by
an excess of fat buildup in the
liver, can result from the
accumulation of visceral fat in the
liver.

• Liver failure and liver cancer are
increased when non-alcoholic
steatohepatitis (NASH) and
cirrhosis, two more serious liver
disorders that can develop from
NAFLD.

7. Apnea during sleep:

The condition known as obstructive sleep apnea, which is characterized by breathing pauses during sleep, is associated with an increased risk of excess abdominal fat.

• Deposits of fat in the neck and throat can restrict airways, causing breathing problems and irregular sleep cycles.

8. Emotional and Psychological Effects:

• Having too much belly fat can have a detrimental effect on one's mental health, body image, and self-esteem. This can result in elevated levels of tension, anxiety, and melancholy.

• Abdominal obesity-related psychological concerns might increase health risks and influence unhealthy lifestyle choices.

Comprehending the health hazards linked to excessive abdominal fat emphasizes the need of implementing lifestyle adjustments to decrease abdominal obesity and enhance general health and wellness.

Chapter Five

The Value of a Well-Balanced Diet

Sufficient Nutrients:

• Eating a balanced diet guarantees that the body gets the right amounts of all vital nutrients, such as vitamins, minerals, protein, carbohydrate, and fats.

• Every nutrient has a distinct function in sustaining biological processes, promoting growth and development, and averting nutritional shortages and related health issues.

2. Energy Balance:

• Eating a balanced diet promotes a healthy energy balance, in which energy expenditure and calorie intake is equal.

• Reaching and maintaining a healthy weight, avoiding weight gain, and lowering the risk of obesity-related disorders all depend on striking a balance between calorie consumption and energy requirements.

3. Maximum Health and Welfare:

• A balanced diet promotes general health and wellbeing by supplying the nutrients required for various body processes, such as immunological response, metabolism, and organ health.

• Foods high in nutrients improve mental and cognitive health, boost tissue growth and repair, and fortify the immune system.

4. Disease Control:

• Lowering the risk of chronic diseases such as heart disease, type 2 diabetes, some malignancies, and osteoporosis can be achieved by eating a balanced diet high in fruits, vegetables, whole grains, lean meats, and healthy fats.

• Antioxidants, phytochemicals, and other bioactive substances included in nutrient-dense diets offer defense against oxidative stress, inflammation, and cellular damage.

5. Weight Control:

• A balanced diet that includes a range of nutrient-dense foods in sensible portion sizes encourages long-term weight management.

• Eating foods high in fiber and in a proportionate amount of fats, proteins, and carbs helps control hunger, encourage fullness, and stop overeating.

6. Gut Health:

• Prebiotic fibers and nutrients that encourage the growth of good gut bacteria are found in a balanced diet, which helps maintain a healthy gut microbiome.

• A varied diet high in whole grains, fruits, vegetables, and fermented foods enhances digestive health and fosters the diversity of the gut flora, which lowers the risk of gastrointestinal illnesses.

7. Life Expectancy and Well-Being:

• A balanced diet is linked to a longer life expectancy and a higher standard of living.

• Good eating practices that are formed early in infancy and continued into maturity enhance general health and vitality by lowering the risk of age-related illnesses and encouraging aging in a healthful manner.

1. **Foods to Include (such
as lean meats, fruits,
veggies, and whole
grains) in order to lose
belly fat**

Yes, without a doubt! Here's
a list of meals that are
especially designed to help
reduce belly fat:

1. Lean Proteins:

• A chicken breast without
skin

• Turkey breast

• Beef cuts that are lean,
such tenderloin or sirloin

• Pork loin

• Fish, particularly oily
varieties such as trout,

salmon, and mackerel

• Shellfish, which includes lobster, crab, and shrimp Tofu and tempeh serve as plant-based alternatives.

• Legumes, such as black beans, chickpeas, and lentils

2. Fruits

• Berries, including blackberries, raspberries, blueberries, and strawberries

• Apples

• Pears

• Oranges

• Grapefruits

• Kiwis

• Watermelon

• Avocado, which is
technically a fruit, for fiber
and good fats

3. Vegetables

• Leafy greens such as
Swiss chard, kale, and
spinach

• vegetables, like Brussels
sprouts, broccoli, and
cauliflower

• Bell peppers, particularly
the vibrant kinds.

• Cucumbers

• Cucumbers

• Zucchini

• Carrots

• Celery

• Garlic with onions

4. Complete Grains:

- Oats, either rolled or steel-cut
- Quinoa
- Brown rice
- Barley

Bulgur

- Products made entirely of wheat (bread, pasta, couscous)
- Buckwheat
- Millet

5. Nutritious Fats:

- Nuts (pistachios, walnuts, and almonds)
- Seeds (pumpkin, chia, and flax seeds)
- Olive oil
- Avocado
- Fatty fish (trout, sardines,

and salmon)

• Nut butters, E.g almond
and peanut butter

**6. Milk and Dairy
Substitutes:**

• Fat-free or low-fat Greek
yogurt

• Low-fat or skim milk

• Cottage cheese (fat-free
or reduced in fat)

• Almond or soy milk
without sugar

**7. Spices, Herbs, and
Additives:**

• Ginger

• Ground cinnamon

• Ginger

• Garlic

• Peppercorns

- Pepper, black
- Herbs for example mint, parsley, cilantro, and basil

8. Water:

- Water (unflavored or flavored with herbs and fruits)
- Herbal teas, including peppermint and green teas
- Sparkling water with a squeeze of lime

When included in a balanced diet, these nutrient-dense, low-calorie, high-protein, high-fiber, and high-healthy-fat foods are great options for encouraging the removal of belly fat.

Food to stay away from or reduce (e.g., sugary beverages, processed foods, saturated fats)

Yes, the following meal list should be restricted or avoided when trying to lose belly fat:

1. Sugar-filled Drinks:

• Cola

• Juices from sweetened fruit

• Energy beverages

• Sweetened coffee and tea beverages

• Sweetened water with extra flavor

2. Foods that have been

processed:

- Contained snacks (cookies, crackers, and chips)
- Sweet cereals for breakfast
- Pre-packaged and frozen dinners
- Fast food (pizza, fries, and hamburgers)
- Processed meats, such as bacon, sausages, and deli meats
- Quick pasta and noodle recipes

3. Fats That Are Saturated:

- Red meat cuts high in fat, like ribeye steaks

- Saturated fat-rich processed meats (such as bacon and sausage)
- Dairy items with added fat (whole milk, cheese, butter)
- Fried food items
- Coconut and palm oils

4. Trans Fats:

- Margarine
- Reducing
- Baked foods and snacks processed using partly hydrogenated oils
- Foods cooked in hydrogenated oils that are fried

5. Excessive Processing of Carbohydrates:

- White bread

- White rice
- Baked dishes and pastries prepared with refined flour
- Sugar-filled cereals
- Instant spaghetti and noodles

6. Added Sugars:

- Candies & confections
- Sweets (ice cream, cakes, and pies)
- Sweet treats (pastries, cookies)
- Dairy items with flavors and sweetened yogurt
- Sugar-added condiments (such as salad dressings, barbecue sauce, and ketchup).

7. Liquor:

- Ale
- Sweetened mixed beverages and cocktails
- Excessive amounts of wine
- Spirits combined with sweeteners

8. Low-Nutrient, High-Calorie Foods:

- Foods high in empty calories, such as candy bars, pretzels, and chips
- snacks with high calorie such as granola bars and trail mix

Instead, concentrate on whole, minimally processed foods that are nutrient-dense and support your weight loss goals.

By cutting back on or avoiding these foods and beverages, you can lower your overall calorie intake, limit the consumption of unhealthy fats and sugars, and create a more conducive environment for belly fat loss.

The importance of mindful and portion control eatiung

1. Control of Portions:

• Portion control helps control calorie intake and avoid overeating by limiting

the quantity of food eaten
at one sitting.

• It enables people to reach
their weight loss objectives
and maintain a balanced
diet while still indulging in a
range of foods.

• People can improve their
relationship with food,
minimize mindless
snacking, and become more
conscious of their eating
patterns by adopting
portion management
practices.

2. Advantages of Controlling Portion:

• Aids in preventing calorie
overload: Reducing portion

sizes helps people avoid ingesting too many calories, which is important for managing their weight and losing belly fat.

• Encourages balanced nutrition: Portion control encourages people to eat a range of foods high in nutrients in sensible amounts, so they get the nutrients they need without going overboard with high-calorie, low-nutrient foods.

• Encourages mindful eating: By paying attention to portion sizes, people can become more aware of their hunger and fullness cues and eat in reaction to their bodies' needs rather than their emotions or their surroundings.

• Helps with weight reduction and maintenance: By encouraging sustainable eating habits and limiting overconsumption, portion control helps prevent weight gain and help create the calorie deficit required for weight loss while maintaining enough nutrition.

3. Portion Control Techniques:

• To visually decrease portion sizes, use smaller

bowls and plates.

• Use kitchen scales,
measuring cups, and spoons
to determine portion sizes.

• Use the "plate method" to
portion your food: half
should be vegetables, 25%
should be lean protein, and
25% should be whole grains
or starchy vegetables.

• Pay attention to the
serving sizes shown on food
packages and follow the
guidelines for portion
amounts.

• Pay attention to your
body's signals of hunger
and fullness, and stop
eating when you're content

rather than too full.

• Take your time, enjoy every bite, and pay attention to the food's flavor, texture, and overall enjoyment.

• To completely enjoy your meal, stay away from distractions like watching TV or using electronics while eating.

4. Intentional Consumption:

• Eating mindfully entails paying close attention to all aspects of the meal, such as the flavor, texture, aroma, and sense of fulfillment it provides.

• It places a strong emphasis on developing a nonjudgmental mindset toward food and eating behaviors, eating with intention and attention, and listening into internal signals of hunger and fullness.

• Emotional eating can be decreased, a person's connection with food can be improved, and eating mindfully can increase one's sense of fulfillment and happiness during meals.

5. Advantages of Intentional Eating:

• Encourages people to
make better food choices:
Mindful eating encourages
people to base their dietary
decisions less on emotional
or environmental cues and
more on internal indicators
of hunger, satiety, and
nutritional needs.

• Promotes greater food
satisfaction and enjoyment:
Mindful eating can promote
greater food satisfaction
and enjoyment by
concentrating on the
sensory aspects of eating,
making meals more
enjoyable.

• Helps with weight

management: Mindful eating can make people more aware of their bodies' signals of hunger and fullness, which helps them avoid overindulging and encourage balanced eating practices that help them lose and maintain weight.

• Lessens stress and emotional eating: attentive eating practices, like attentive awareness and deep breathing, can assist people in managing stress and lessen the chance that they will resort to food for solace or emotional support.

6. Useful Advice for

Mindful Eating:

• Savor every bite of food by chewing it well and eating slowly.

• Be mindful of your body's signals of hunger and fullness; eat when you're hungry and stop when you're full.

• Observe food-related thoughts and feelings without passing judgment, and note impulses or cravings without acting on them right away.

• Develop an attitude of thankfulness for the sustenance that food provides, savoring the

tastes, textures, and
nutrients in every meal.

• Use all of your senses
when eating, taking note of
the flavors, textures, colors,
and scents of the food as
well as the sounds and
feelings associated with it.
People can support their
weight reduction and
general well-being
objectives, foster better
digestion and nutrient
absorption, and create
healthy eating habits by
adopting portion
management and mindful
eating practices into their

everyday lives.

Chapter Six

Exercises That Are Good for Targeting Belly Fat

1. Exercise for the Heart:

• Cardio exercises help reduce body fat overall, including belly fat, by raising heart rate and calorie expenditure.

• Cardio exercises that involve brisk walking, jogging, cycling, swimming, and jumping rope are beneficial.

• For maximum fat-burning

advantages, aim for at least 150 minutes of moderate-intensity or 75 minutes of vigorous-intensity cardio every week.

2. Strengthening Exercise:

• Strength training, which results in muscle growth, can speed up metabolism and encourage the reduction of fat, including visceral fat.

• Exercises that combine several muscular groups, such lunges, dead lifts, bench presses, and squats, are very beneficial.

• Include two to three times a week resistance training sessions with an emphasis on gradually stressing muscles with larger weights or more resistance.

3. HIIT, or high-intensity interval training:

• HIIT workouts efficiently burn calories and promote fat reduction by alternating short bursts of intense exercise with rest intervals.

• For a full body workout, mix activities like sprints, burpees, jumping jacks, and mountain climbers into your HIIT circuits.

• Because of the after burn effect, HIIT sessions can be finished faster than conventional cardio workouts and continue to burn calories afterward.

4. Fundamental Exercises:

• Focused core exercises help to create a tighter, more defined waistline by strengthening abdominal muscles and enhancing core stability.

• To work the rectus abdominis, obliques, and transverse abdominis muscles, incorporate movements like planks, crunches, Russian twists, bicycle crunches, and leg raises.

• Include a range of core exercises in your workouts two to three times a week, paying close attention to form and technique to get the most out of them.

5. Training in intervals:

• By alternating between periods of high-intensity exercise and low-intensity recuperation, interval training significantly increases fat burning and metabolism.

• Use interval circuits that combine strength and aerobic training to target belly fat and build lean muscle at the same time.

• Boot camp-style sessions, Tabata exercises, and circuit training are a few examples of interval training.

6.Exercises for Flexibility and Mobility:

• By increasing flexibility, lowering muscular tension, and improving overall movement quality, stretching and mobility exercises make workouts more efficient.

• Use static stretches to cool down after exercise and dynamic stretches and mobility drills to warm up before.

• Yoga and Pilates programs combine exercises for strengthening the core with flexibility, offering a comprehensive strategy for reducing belly fat and enhancing general fitness.

7.Regularity and Increasing Overload:

• The secret to reaching and maintaining fat loss objectives is consistency in exercise, no matter what kind it is.

• Gradually raise the duration, frequency, and intensity of your workouts over time to keep your body challenged and prevent plateaus.

• Use a variety of exercise techniques to target belly fat from several perspectives, keep sessions interesting, and avoid boredom.

Adding extra exercise to one's everyday routine (e.g., walking, taking the stairs)

Exercise regimens are not the only option to add additional physical activity to your daily life. Simple lifestyle adjustments and finding opportunities to move more throughout the day can build up and improve one's overall health and physical fitness. Increasing physical activity in daily life can be achieved in the following ways:

1. Walking:

• during your breaks from work or school, go for a quick stroll.

• To add extra steps, park further away from your destination.

• For quick excursions, cycle or walk rather than drive.

• Set and monitor daily step targets with a pedometer or fitness tracker.

2. Getting Up the Steps:

• whenever feasible, it's advisable to use the stairs over the elevator.

• For an added workout, push

yourself to ascend stairs quickly
or to take two steps at a time.

3. Active commuting:

• Use public transportation or
walk or bike instead of driving to
work.

• Stand rather than sit when
taking public transportation to
strengthen your legs and enhance
your balance.

4. Domestic Tasks:

• Take advantage of housework
as an opportunity to exercise.

• Use intense motions to dust,
mop, vacuum, and raise heart
rate in order to burn calories.

• Yard and garden tasks like
weeding and grass mowing can
also be quite beneficial to your

fitness.

5. Playtime with pets and family:

• Play outdoor sports like soccer, Frisbee, or tag with your family or pets to spend active time together.

• Walk or trek with your dog on a regular basis to maintain your health and fitness levels.

6. Engaging Recreational Activities:

• Take part in enjoyable leisure pursuits, such hiking, swimming, dancing, or sports.

• To meet new people and maintain your motivation, sign up for a fitness class or local sports league.

7. Standing and Intermittent Movement:

• Get up and stretch frequently, particularly if you lead a sedentary lifestyle or work.

• Use a timer to remind yourself to get up and move a little bit during the day.

8. Enhancements for the Home:

• Make small changes to your home's layout to promote movement, including moving furniture to make more room for stretches and workouts.

• For easy workouts, purchase home exercise equipment like dumbbells or resistance bands.

Chapter seven

Techniques for managing stress and their effect on abdominal fat

By addressing the underlying causes of abdominal obesity, stress management approaches are essential in the reduction of abdominal fat. Persistent stress causes the body to react physiologically, which may encourage the buildup of visceral fat and raise the risk of metabolic issues and associated health issues. Reducing these impacts and promoting belly fat loss can be achieved by putting into practice efficient stress management strategies. The following stress-reduction methods and how they affect abdominal fat:

1.Meditation with mindfulness:

• Mindfulness meditation, which helps ease tension and encourage relaxation, entails focusing attention on the present moment without passing judgment.

• Studies indicate that consistent mindfulness training can enhance

general metabolic health,
decrease cortisol levels, and
reduce belly fat.

2. Breathing Techniques:

• Deep breathing techniques,
such diaphragmatic or belly
breathing, lower stress hormone
levels and trigger the body's
relaxation response.

• Regularly engaging in deep
breathing exercises can help
decrease cortisol levels, ease
tension, and prevent the buildup
of belly fat caused by stress.

3. PMR, or progressive muscle relaxation, is:

PMR is a methodical way to
produce deep relaxation by
tensing and relaxing various

muscle groups.

• Regular PMR practice lowers the risk of belly obesity by promoting relaxation, easing stress, and reducing muscle tension.

4. Yoga:

• Yoga encourages relaxation and stress alleviation by combining physical postures, breathing exercises, and meditation. Regular yoga practice has been linked to lower cortisol levels, improved insulin sensitivity, and a decrease in visceral fat, or belly fat.

5. Frequent Workout:

• Exercise is a potent stress reliever that can counteract the detrimental effects of ongoing stress on the buildup of abdominal fat.

• Regular exercise, such as yoga, strength training, or cardio, lowers cortisol levels, produces endorphins, and enhances general wellbeing. All of these benefits can help with the reduction of belly fat.

6.Good Living Practices:

• Developing healthy lifestyle practices that promote stress reduction and belly fat loss include getting enough sleep, eating a balanced diet, and abstaining from alcohol.

• Setting limits, prioritizing self-care tasks, and using time management techniques can all help lower stress levels and improve general health.

7.Social Assistance:

• Building strong social ties and asking friends, family, or support groups for assistance can help provide emotional support and mitigate the negative effects of stress on the buildup of belly fat.

• Developing strong relationships, spending time with loved ones, and participating in meaningful activities can all help people become more resilient to stress and feel better overall.

It is possible to effectively lower stress levels, lessen the detrimental effects of ongoing stress on the buildup of belly fat, and support your efforts to reach and maintain a healthy weight and lifestyle by implementing these stress management tactics into your daily routine.

Techniques for sustaining weight loss and avoiding the return of abdominal fat

1.Regular Exercise Schedule:
• Keep up your normal exercise regimen to help you maintain your weight and avoid gaining back belly fat.
To improve general fitness and metabolic health, try to incorporate cardiovascular,

strength, and core activities.

• To maintain long-term results and motivation, find activities you enjoy and include them into your routine on a regular basis.

2.Optimal Eating Practices:

• Keep a diet that is well-balanced and full of whole, nutrient-dense foods including whole grains, fruits, vegetables, lean meats, and healthy fats.

• Manage your portions, eat mindfully, and use your intuition when eating to prevent overindulging and make informed dietary decisions that will help you maintain your weight.

• identify the situations that lead to emotional eating and seek out healthy eating method like journaling, physical activity, or methods of relaxation.

3. Consistent observation and responsibility:

• To assess your progress and see any possible obstacles, keep a regular eye on your weight, body measurements, and food intake.

• To measure your calorie intake, macronutrient balance, and eating habits, keep a food journal or utilize a monitoring app.

• Be responsible for your actions by establishing reasonable objectives, asking friends or a support group for help, and acknowledging your accomplishments along the way.

4.Stress Reduction and Self-Taking:

• Give stress-reduction methods like yoga, deep breathing exercises, mindfulness meditation, or relaxation techniques top priority in order to lower stress levels and stop stress-related weight gain in the abdomen.

• Engage in self-care routines that encourage calm and wellbeing, such as getting enough sleep, going outside, engaging in hobbies, and spending time with close friends and family.

5. Behavioral Techniques and the Development of Habits:

- Recognize and deal with any potential stressors or barriers to maintaining a healthy weight, such as social expectations, emotional eating, or boredom.
- Create constructive coping techniques and substitute methods to handle stress, boredom, or unpleasant feelings without turning to food.
- Rather than relying on restricted diets or quick cures, put your attention on creating long-lasting habits and lifestyle adjustments that promote long-term health and wellbeing.

6. Frequent Self-Evaluation and Modification:

- Regularly evaluate your

progress, pinpoint any areas that need work, and make the required dietary, activity, or behavioral changes.

• Be versatile and flexible in your approach, understanding that maintaining your weight calls for constant work and modifications to account for evolving demands and situations.

Chapter Eight

Inspiration for readers to continue on their own path

Of course! It might be difficult to start a journey toward improved health and wellness, which includes losing weight and reducing belly fat, but it can also be very rewarding. Here are some

words of wisdom for readers
embarking on their own journey:

**1.Honor each and every win,
no matter how small:**

• Remind yourself to acknowledge
and appreciate each small victory
along the path, such as reaching
a goal for weight loss, choosing
better foods, or maintaining your
workout schedule. No matter how
tiny, every advancement is a step
in the right direction.

**2. Treat Yourself with
Kindness:**

• throughout your journey, it is
imperative that you treat yourself
with kindness and care.
Remember that everything is a
part of the process, even though

there may be obstacles or frustrating times. Always be nice and understanding to yourself just as you would to a friend in a similar position.

3. Put Progress First Rather than Perfection:

• Aim for advancement rather than perfection. It's acceptable to experience imperfect days or instances in which plans don't work out. The most important thing is that you are determined to change for the better and advance step by step.

4. Have faith in your fortitude and resiliency:

• You underestimate your strength and resiliency. Have

faith in your capacity to overcome barriers, endure hardships, and accomplish your objectives. Have faith in your own abilities to develop and change.

5.Accept the Journey:

• Keep in mind that your path to health and wellness is about more than just getting where you're going; it's also about the experiences, insights, and personal development you have along the way. Accept the trip, relish every second, and be grateful for the chance to make an investment in your health.

6. Remain Steady and Unwavering:

• Perseverance and consistency

are essential for success in any undertaking. Remain dedicated to your objectives in spite of challenges or disappointments. Continue taking care of yourself, choosing good decisions, and moving in the direction of a better, healthier life.

Resources and instruments for monitoring development (e.g., food journal, fitness apps)

A vital component of any path towards health and wellbeing, including the decrease of belly fat and weight loss, is monitoring progress. Thankfully, there are lots of tools and resources out there to support you in tracking your development and maintaining responsibility. The following are some useful instruments and sources for monitoring advancement:

1.Journal of Food:

• You can monitor your daily intake of meals, snacks, and drinks by keeping a food journal. You can keep track of the kinds of food you eat, how much you eat, and any situational or emotional circumstances that might affect your eating patterns.

• There are options for keeping a food journal that are both digital and physical, such as websites, apps, and paper notebooks.

Decide on a method that suits you the most, then make a commitment to regularly logging your meals.

2. Fitness Applications:

• You may monitor your progress toward your objectives, exercise, diet, and other elements of your health and fitness with the use of fitness applications.

• Well-known fitness applications include Lose It! and MyFitnessPal, and Fit bit let you record your food intake, keep tabs on your exercise, make goals, and track your development over time. To assist you in staying on track, a lot of these applications also include functions like meal planning, calorie counting, and social support.

3. Fitness trackers that are wearable:

• Real-time data on heart rate, sleep habits, physical activity, and other topics can be obtained from wearable fitness trackers, such as fitness bands or smart watches.

• Tracking steps, distance, calories burnt, and active minutes throughout the day with devices like Fitbit, Garmin, and Apple Watch provides information on your total activity level and advancement toward fitness objectives.

4. Body Measurements and

Developmental Images:

• Monitoring physical attributes like weight, waist size, and body fat % can reveal important information about how the body's composition changes over time.

• Take frequent progress shots from various viewpoints to visibly monitor your body's changes and recognize your accomplishments along the road.

5.Websites promoting health and wellness:

• There are a plethora of tools and resources available on health and wellness-focused online platforms and websites for monitoring progress, getting instructional content, and interacting with a supportive community.

• You can stay informed and inspired along your journey by using the articles, tools, calculators, and forums found on websites like Spark People, Health line, and Very well fit.